THE BIGGER PICTURE

ROBERT HANCOCK

ISBN: 979-8-9911338-0-7 (Paperback)
       979-8-9911338-1-4 (E-book)

Library of Congress Control Number: 2024915093

Published By:

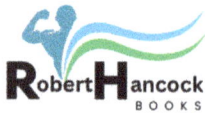

Pittsburg CA, 94565
https://www.robert-hancock.org/

Publisher Provider:

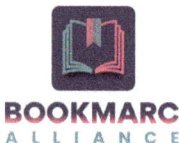

BOOKMARC
ALLIANCE

This manual will benefit Uber drivers, Lyft drivers, Truck operators, Highway Patrol, Bus operators, and those that sit for a living.

Robert T. Hancock

Nationally Certified Personal Trainer w/ American Council on Exercise T162139,

Older Adult Fitness Specialist w/ Exercise, etc. #1806605 & City Bus Operator for 25 years and counting.

I'm available for demonstrations & lectures. Robthancock@gmail.com

Photos by Jasmine Nicole Hancock Publishing: Coach Kadija Philips

Much appreciation to Typing Services for their excellent typing skills and great patience.

Table of Contents

Hi,

Thank you for making health your priority. My name is Robert Troy Hancock. I am a city bus operator with 25 years of experience and counting. As a bus operator for 25 years, I know the negative effects of driving for a living. I am a Nationally Certified Personal Trainer with the American Council on Exercise (since 2012) as well as an Older Adult Fitness Specialist with Exercise etc. (since 2018). With that experience and knowledge, I know a few things about how to fight off the negative effects of driving for a living.

In this manual, I explain the muscles that are affected when driving/ sitting for long durations. I also demonstrate how to exercise those muscles. In addition, there are tips in regard to healthy living for commercial drivers, which will contribute toward longevity in their careers as commercial drivers.

Hip Flexors

The purpose of hip flexors is to bring the legs up to the torso. They are flexed when sitting. Tight hip flexors contribute to back problems.

When driving, commercial drivers have their hip flexors flexed. When they leave the driver's seat, their backs have challenges getting back to an erect position. Years of driving can eventually cause a bent-over walking posture for an operator.

One of the remedies for a bent-over walking posture is to stretch your hip flexors throughout the day as well as at the end of the day. Another way to stretch hip flexors is by walking in reverse. Walking in reverse involves more hip extension than flexion.

Hamstrings

The hamstrings are the posterior thigh muscles. They are responsible for the flexion of the knee and extension of the hip. When sitting, hamstrings flex and are likely to get tight if not stretched regularly. Tight hamstrings can cause back problems as well as knee problems.

Sitting over an hour without stretching every hour will really tighten up the hamstrings. After an hour, the operator should exit the seat and reach for his or her toes without bending the knees. You should not bounce with the stretch. Reach for your toes and hold the position for at least 30 seconds.

Quadriceps

The quadriceps are the anterior thigh muscles. They are responsible for the extension of the knee and the flexion of the hip.

Excessive sitting weakens the quadriceps and may lead to knee problems.

Imbalance due to one's sitting position can cause injuries. The imbalance develops from sitting for too long with the knee flexed without extending. That compromises the knee's stability.

To overcome or avoid the problem, it is important to get out of the seat and extend your knees by walking after every hour of driving.

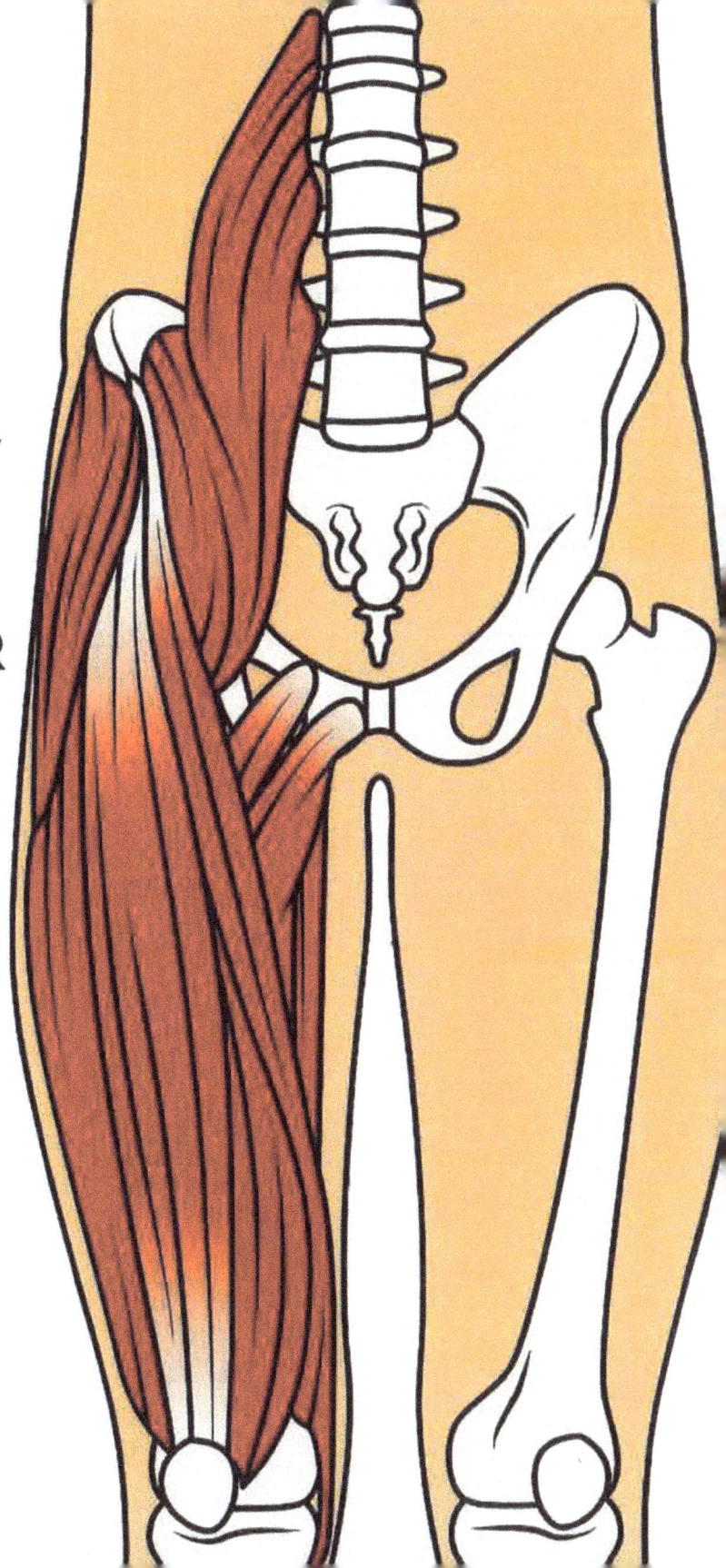

HIP FLEXOR

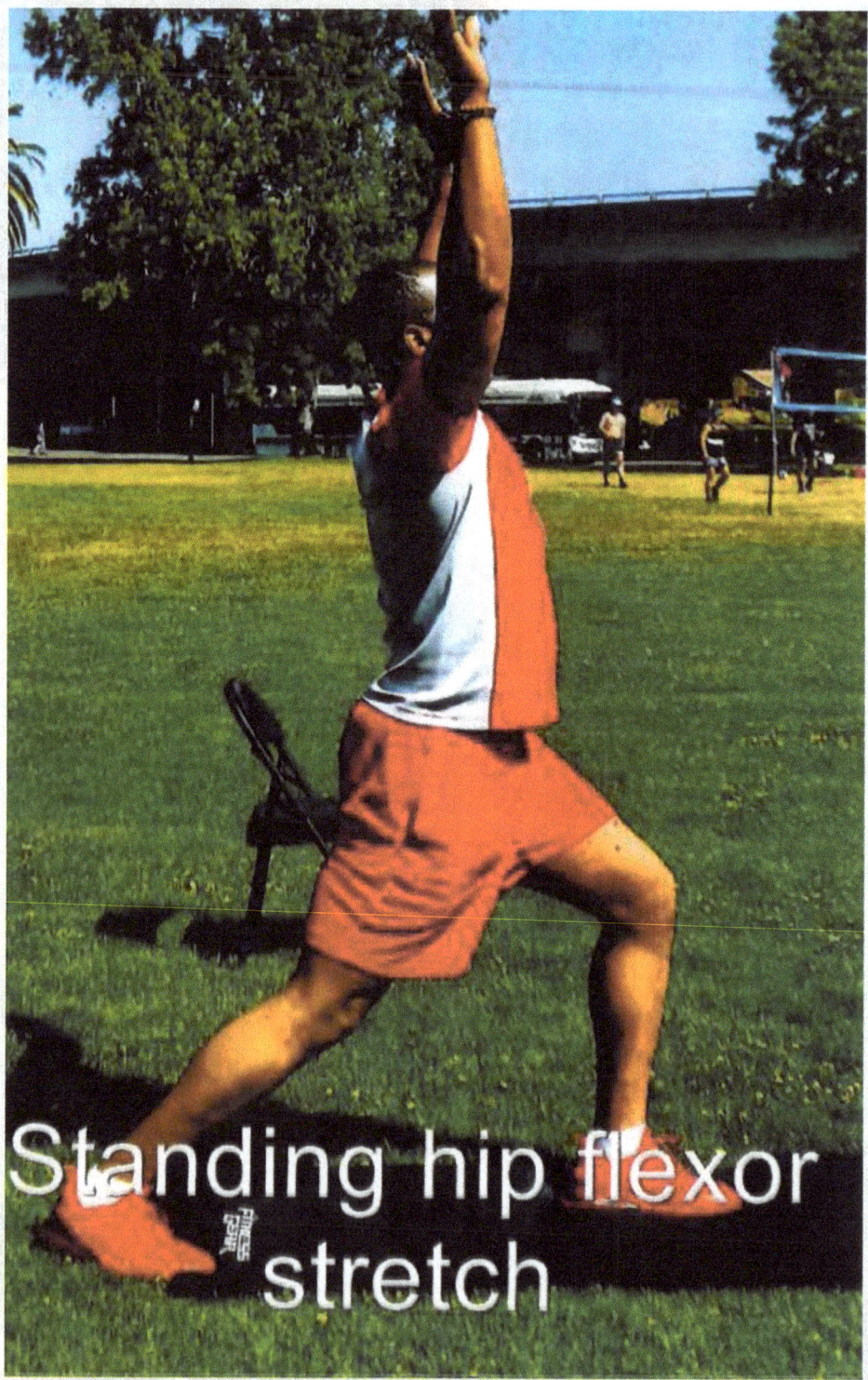

Standing hip flexor stretch

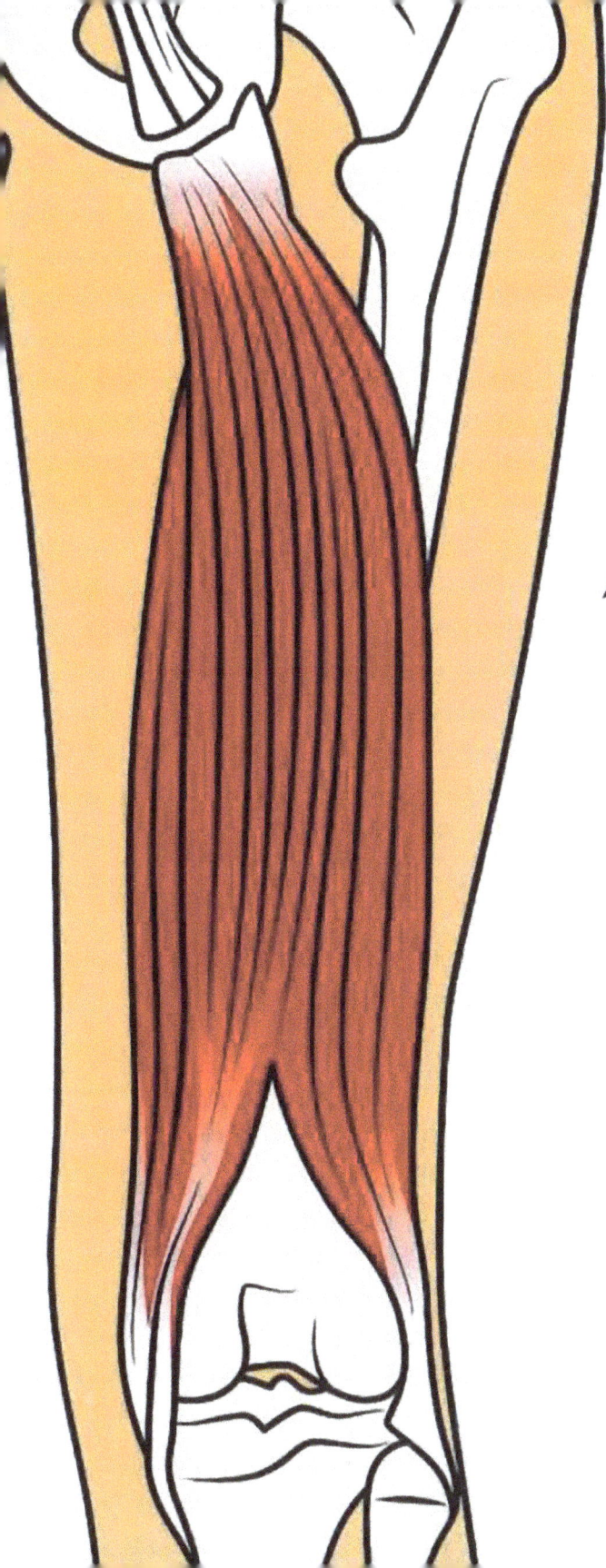
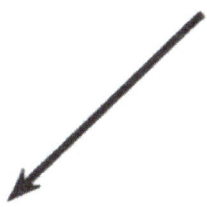

HAMSTRING

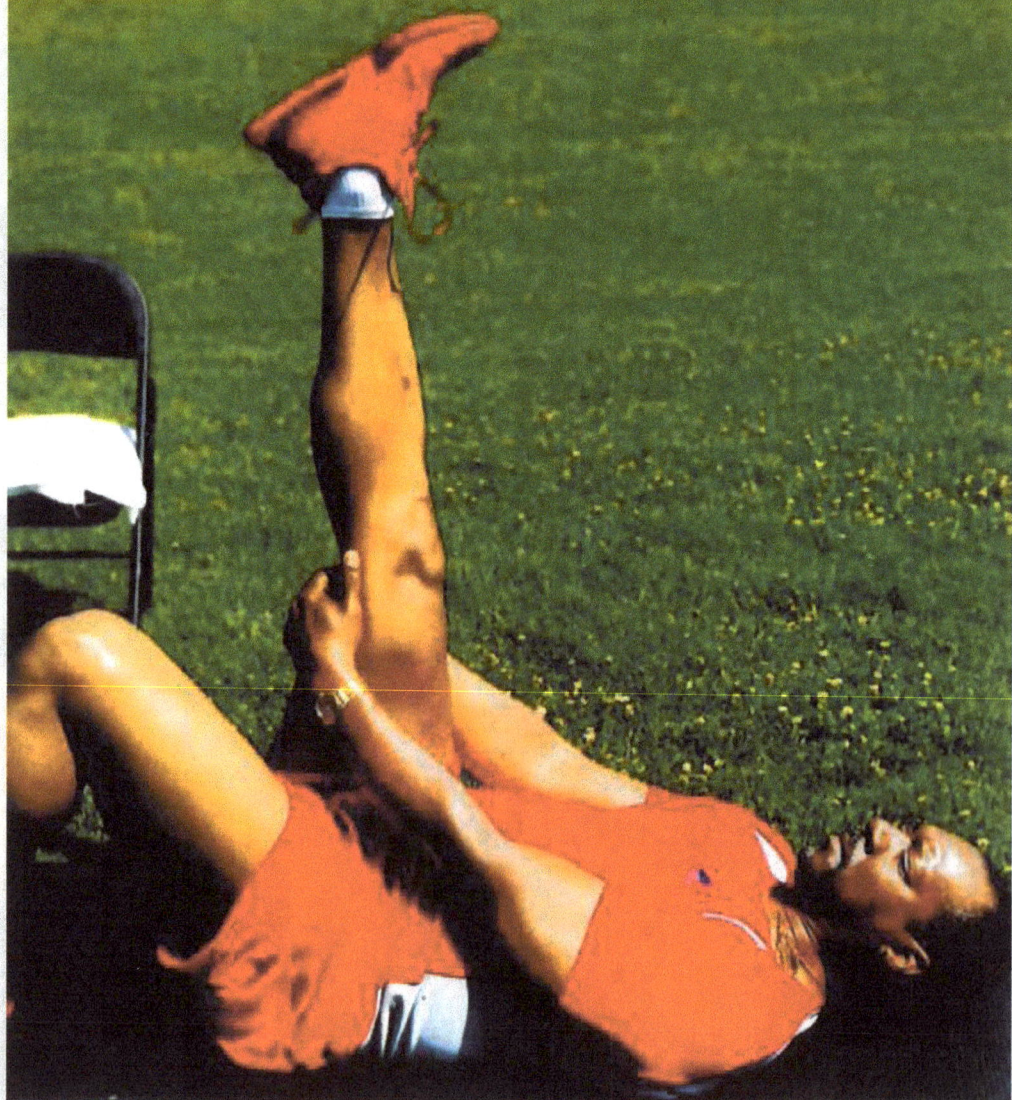

Hamstring stretch

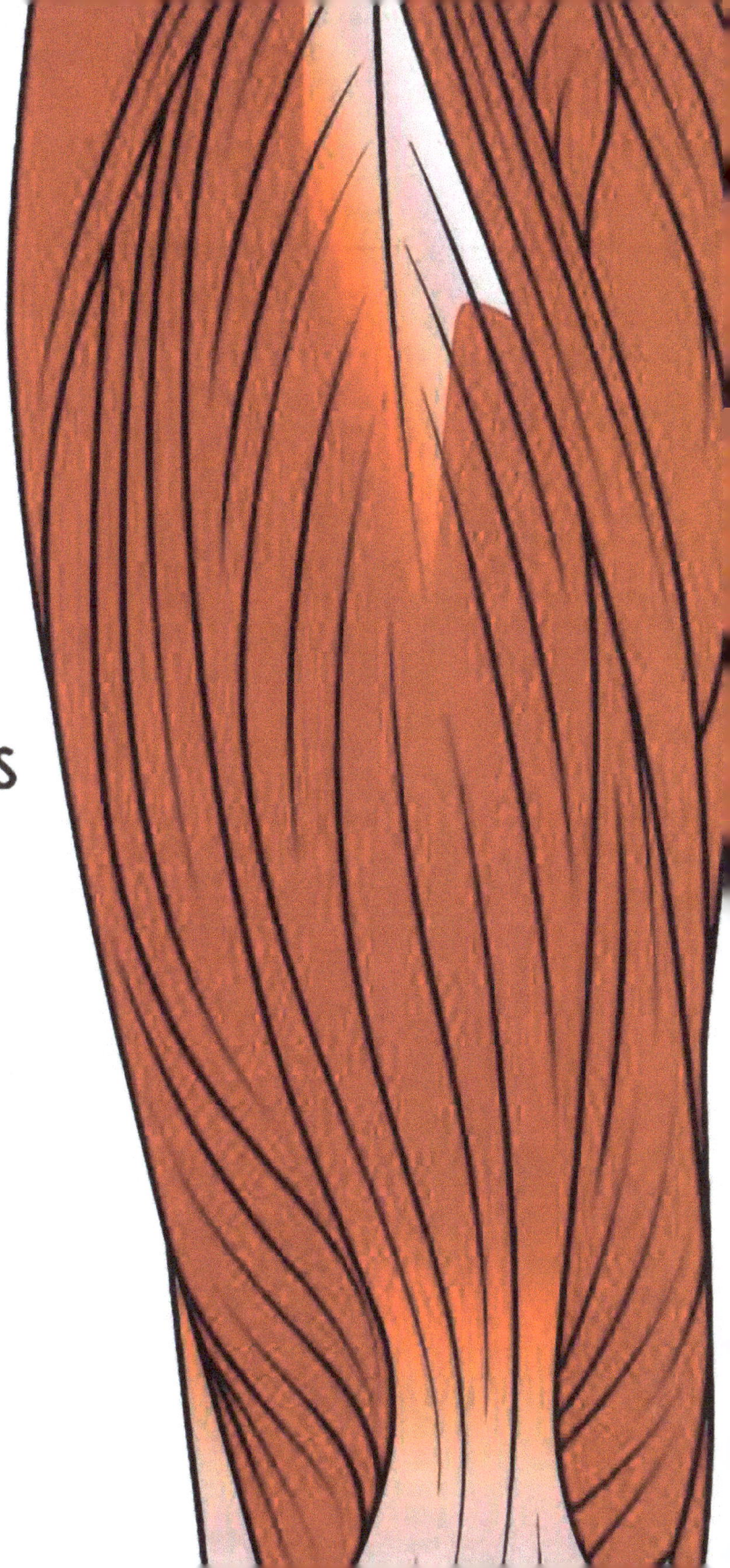

JADRICEPS

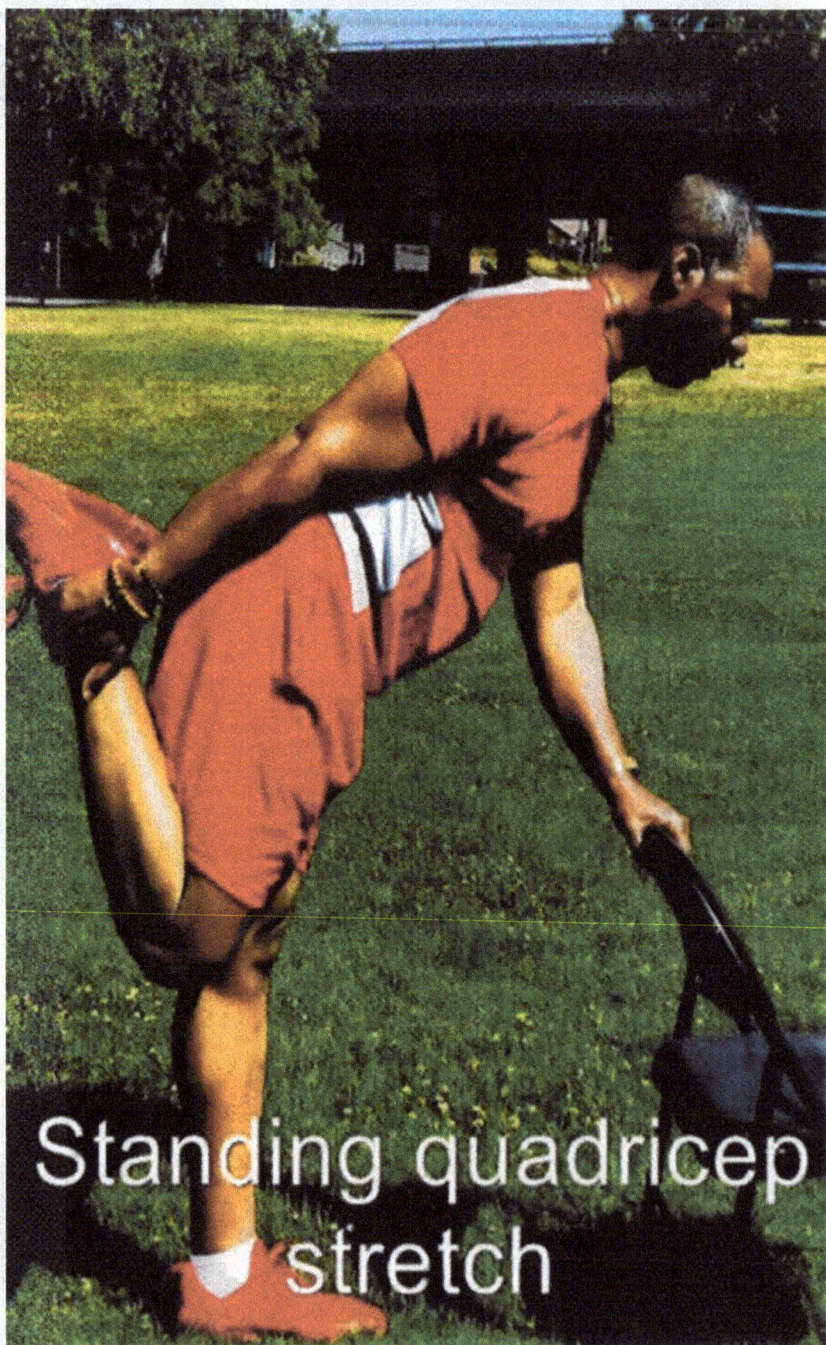

Standing quadricep stretch

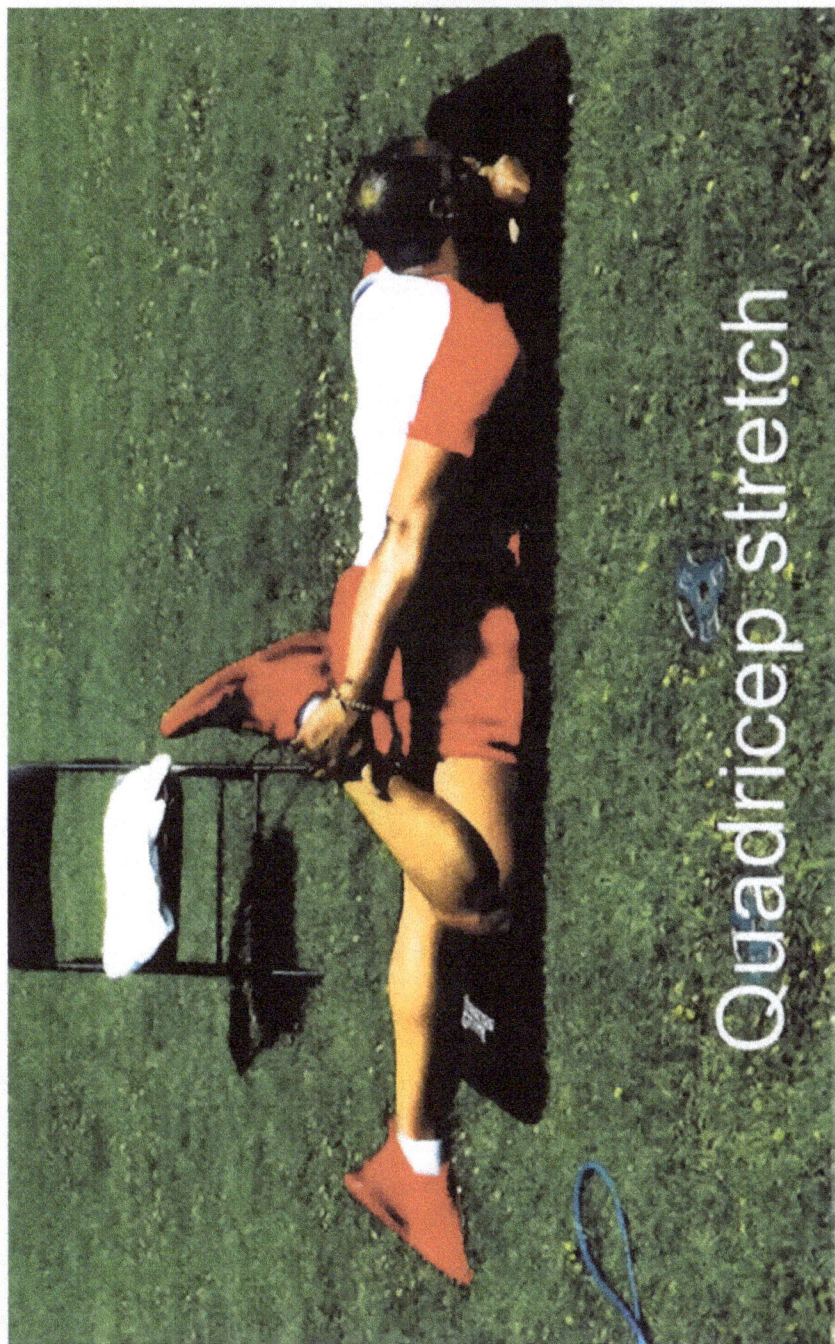

Quadricep stretch

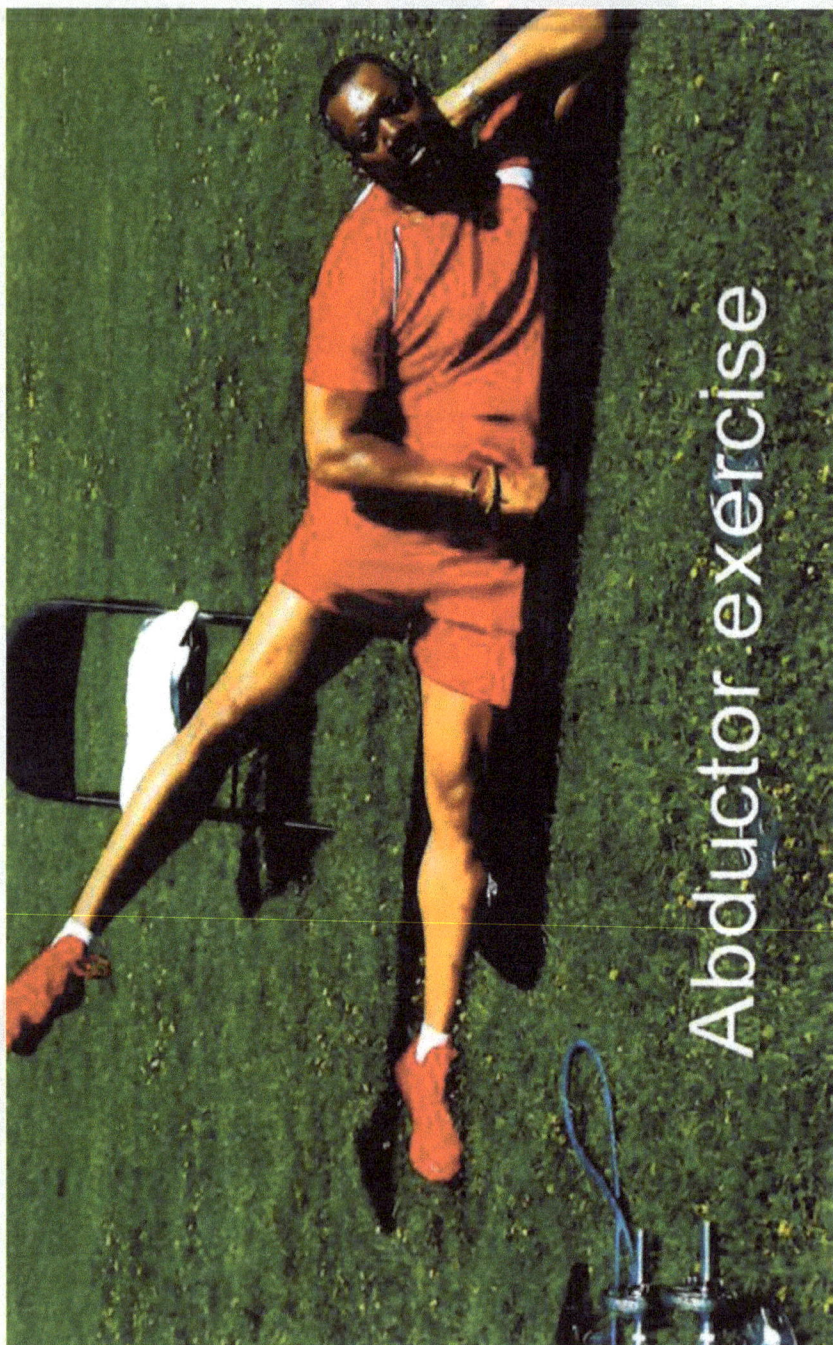

Abductor exercise

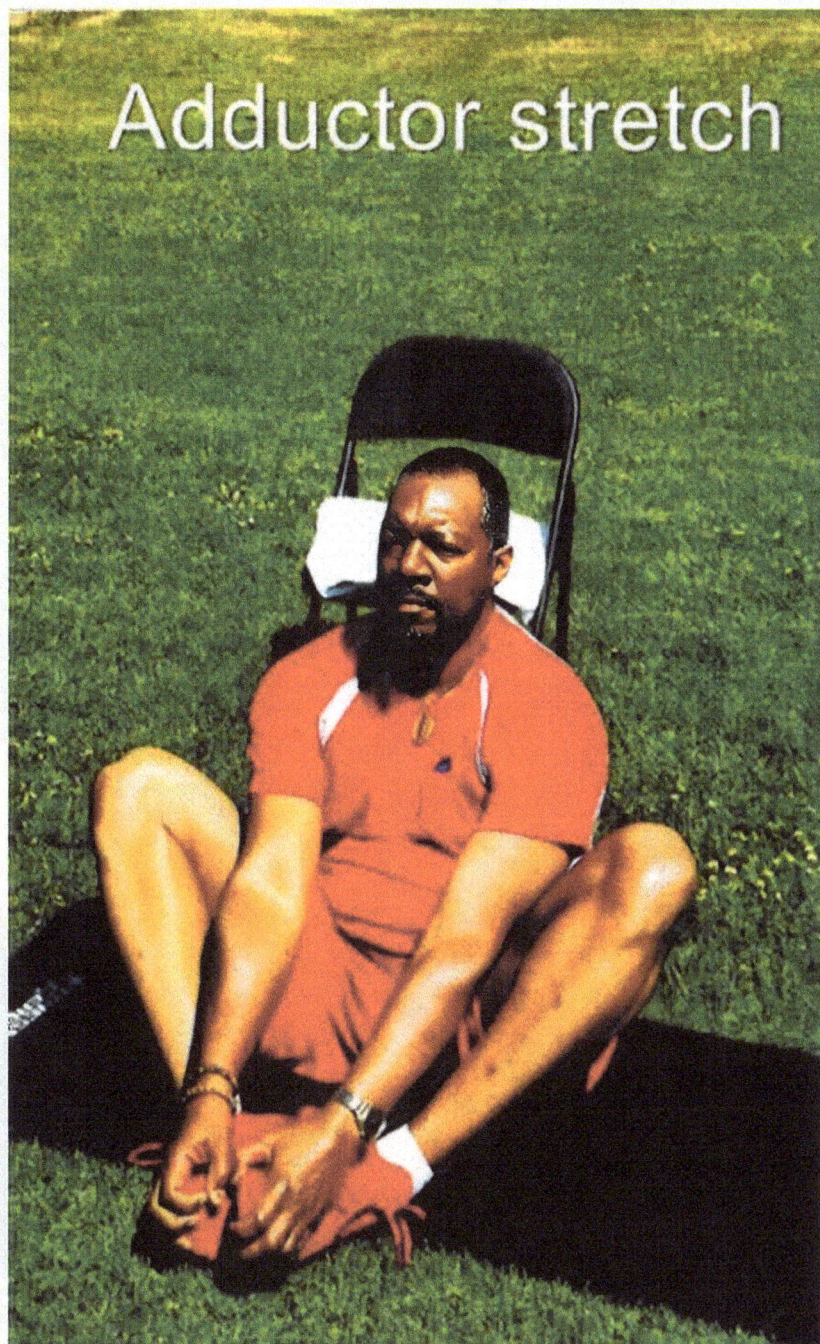

Adductor stretch

Achilles Tendon

The Achilles tendon connects the calf muscle to the heel bone. Pain in the Achilles tendon can occur after long periods of sitting. One may also experience tight calf muscles.

To avoid issues with the Achilles tendon, you need to get out of the seat and stretch your Achilles tendon after driving for an hour.

A ruptured Achilles tendon requires months of rehabilitation and rest.

Glutes

The glutes are the butt muscles. They work anytime you raise your thigh to the side, rotate your leg, or thrust your hips forward. The extension of the hip also activates the glutes.

Constant sitting weakens the glutes. It also tightens the hip flexors. Muscle weakness can pull or pinch nerves, causing numbness. Underused glutes can cause back problems.

To minimize problems with your glutes, you need to get out of the seat and do some squats (if possible) or find some stairs to climb after every hour of driving. Lunges are also a good exercise for the glutes. Walking an incline (hill) also targets the glutes.

Deltoids

The deltoids are shoulder muscles responsible for the lifting and rotation of the arm. They are used quite a bit when driving. When driving, mostly the front and side parts of the shoulder are active. The rear shoulders do not get much work when driving. As a result, there is an imbalance, which is responsible for pain and injury to the shoulder.

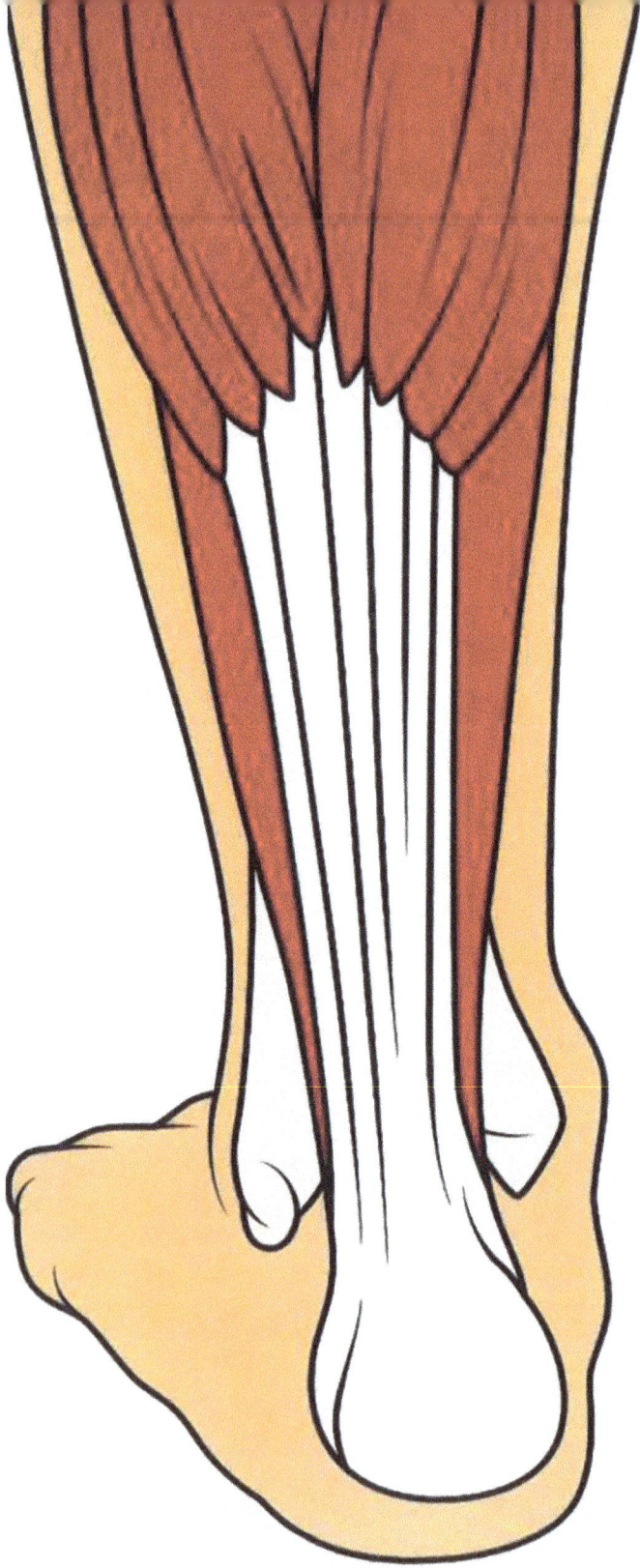

ACHILLE
TENDON

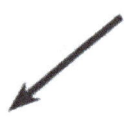

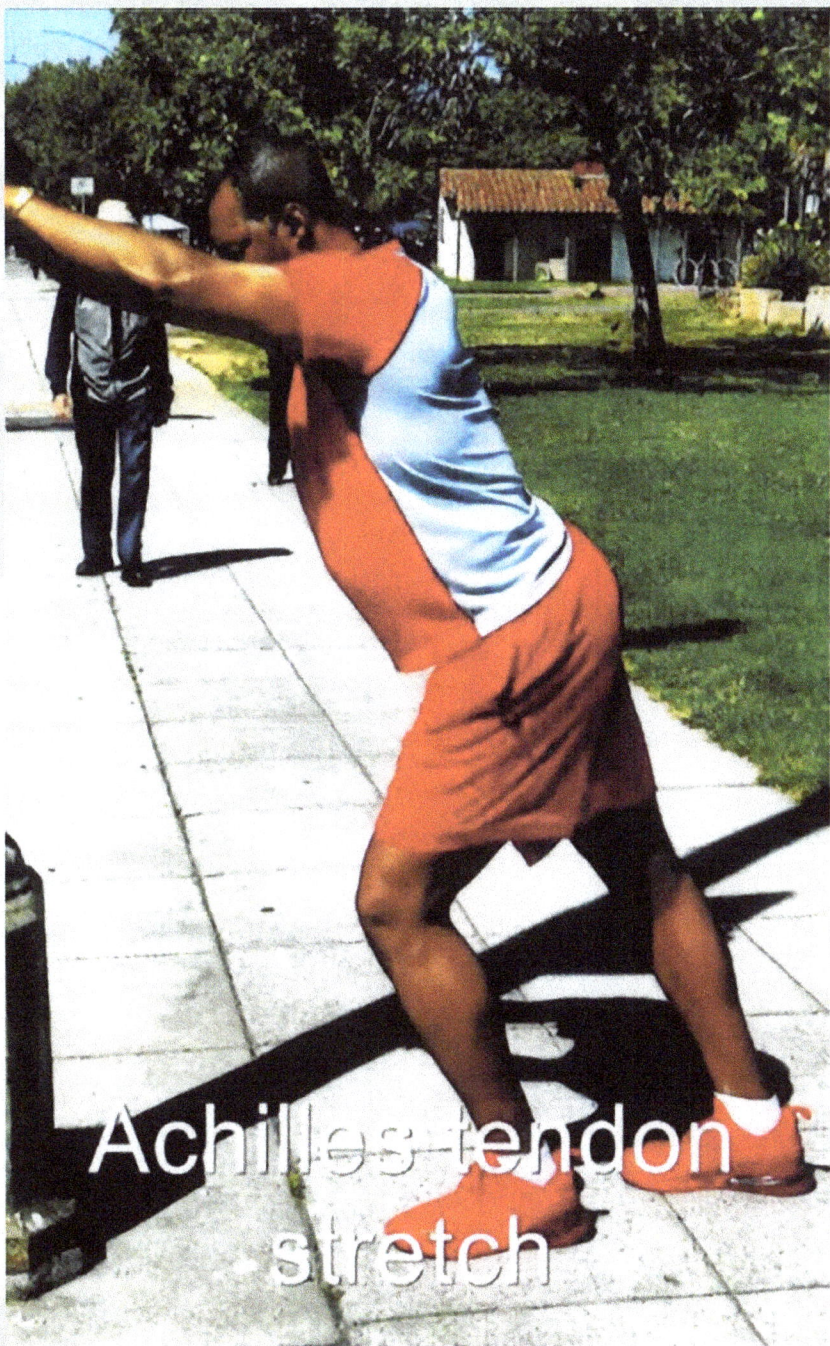

Achilles tendon stretch

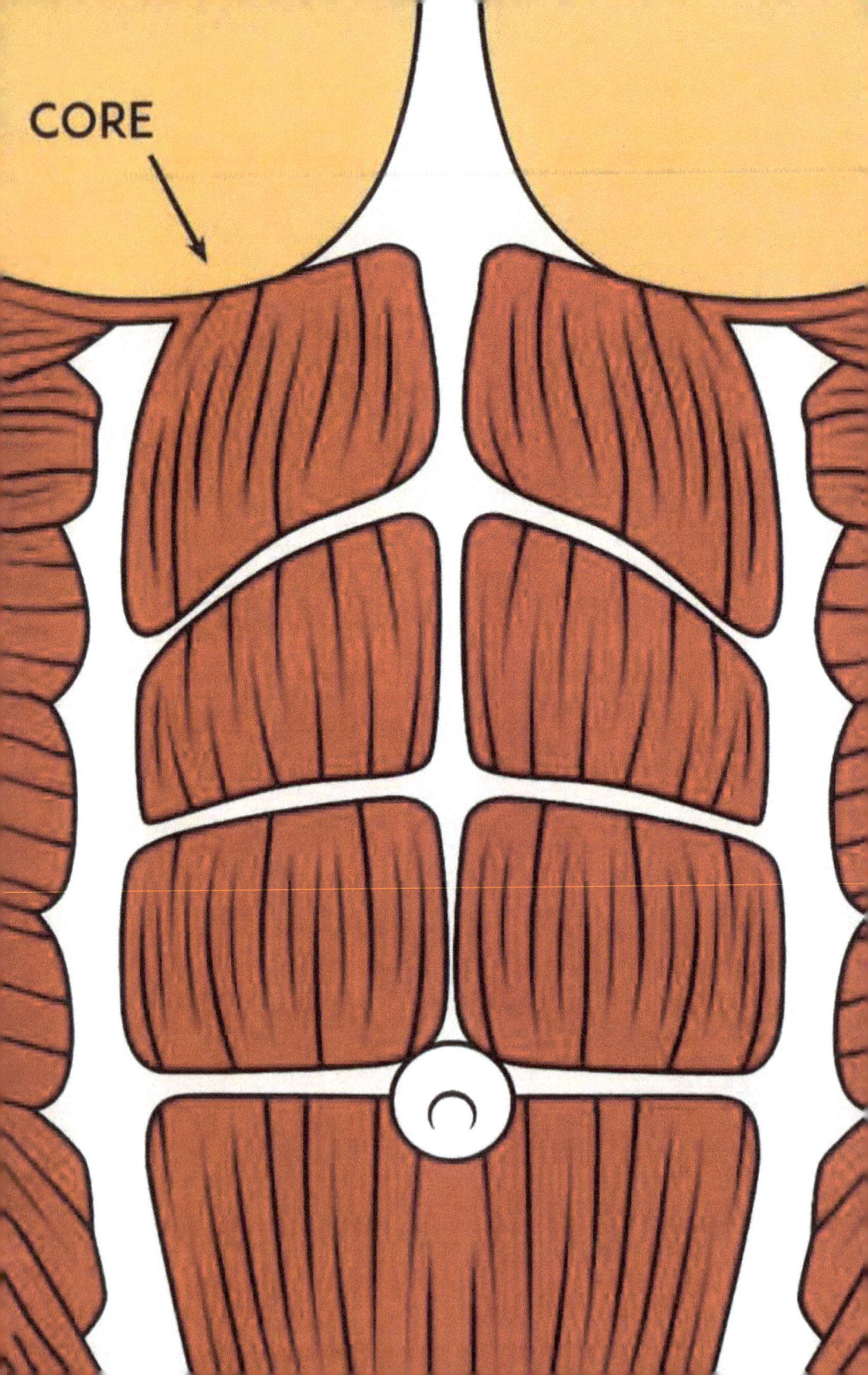

CORE

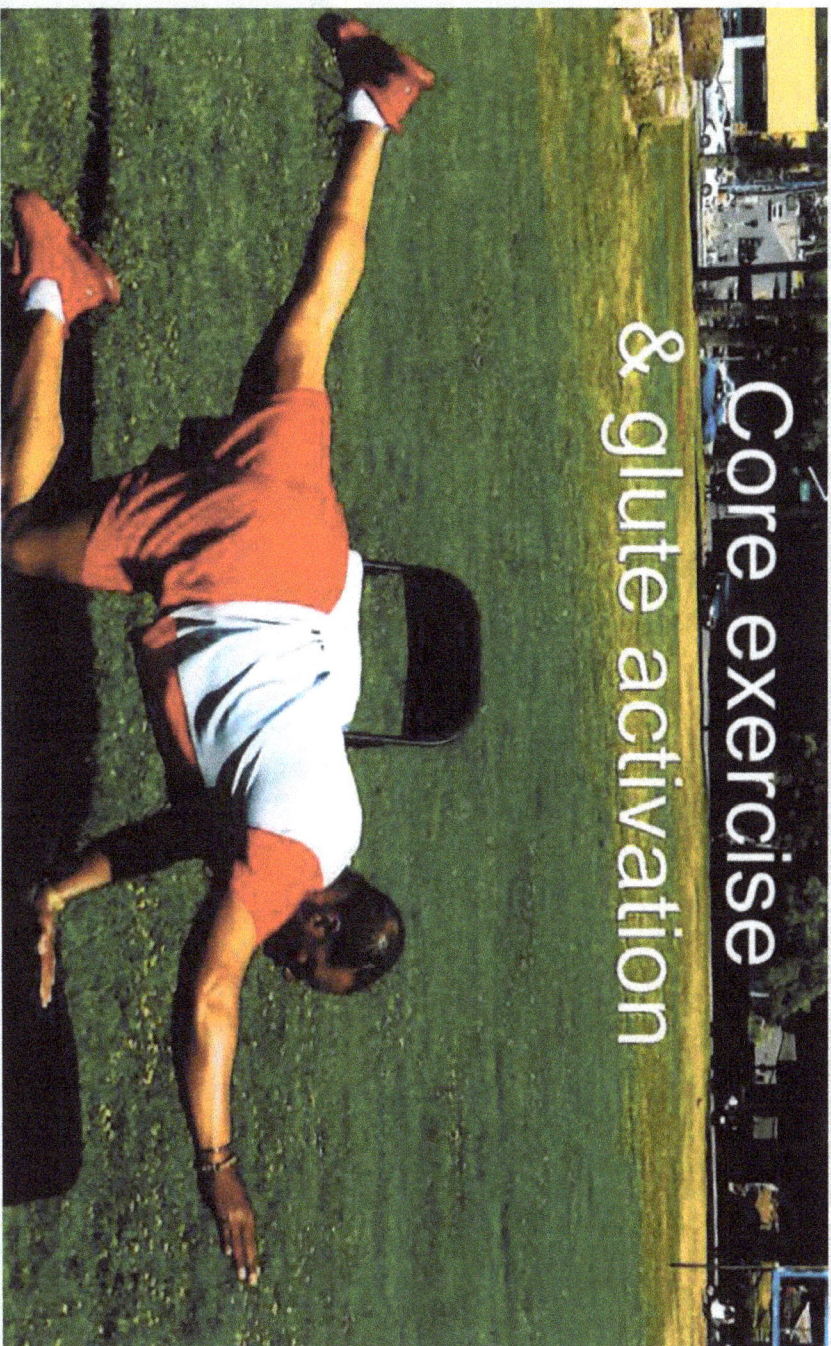
Core exercise & glute activation

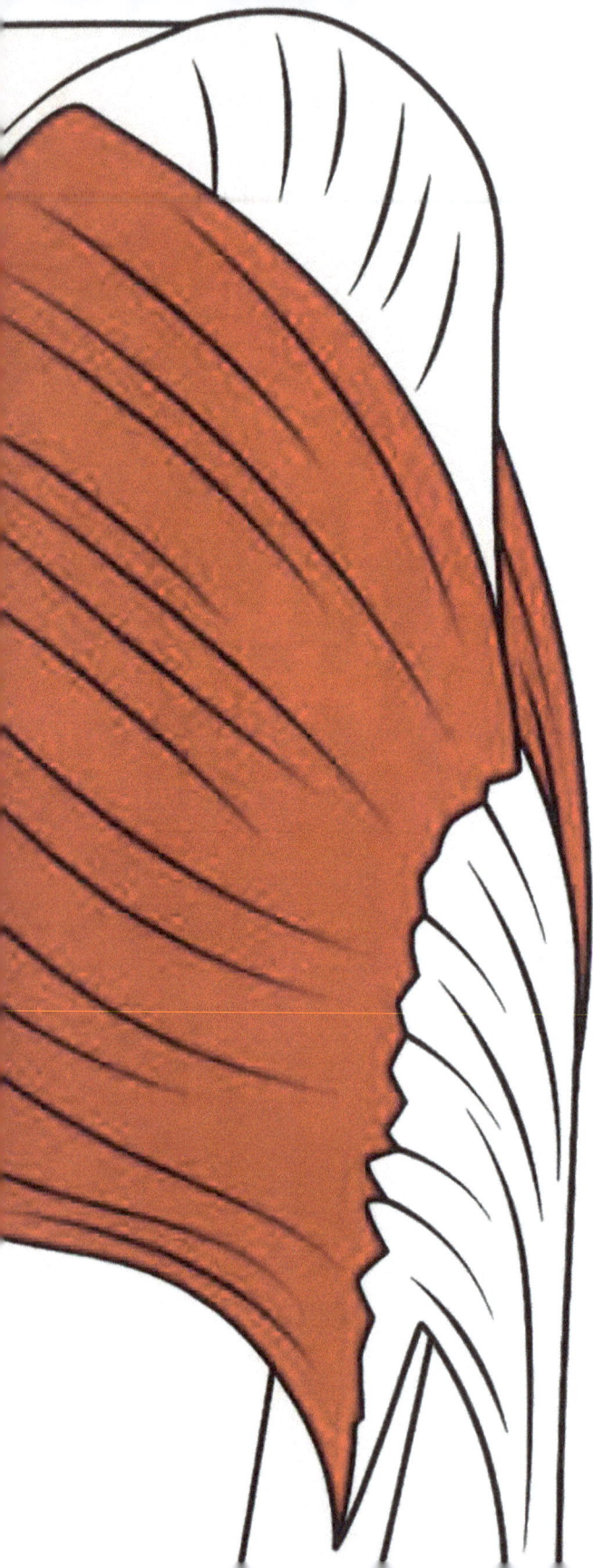

GLUTE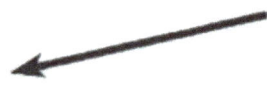

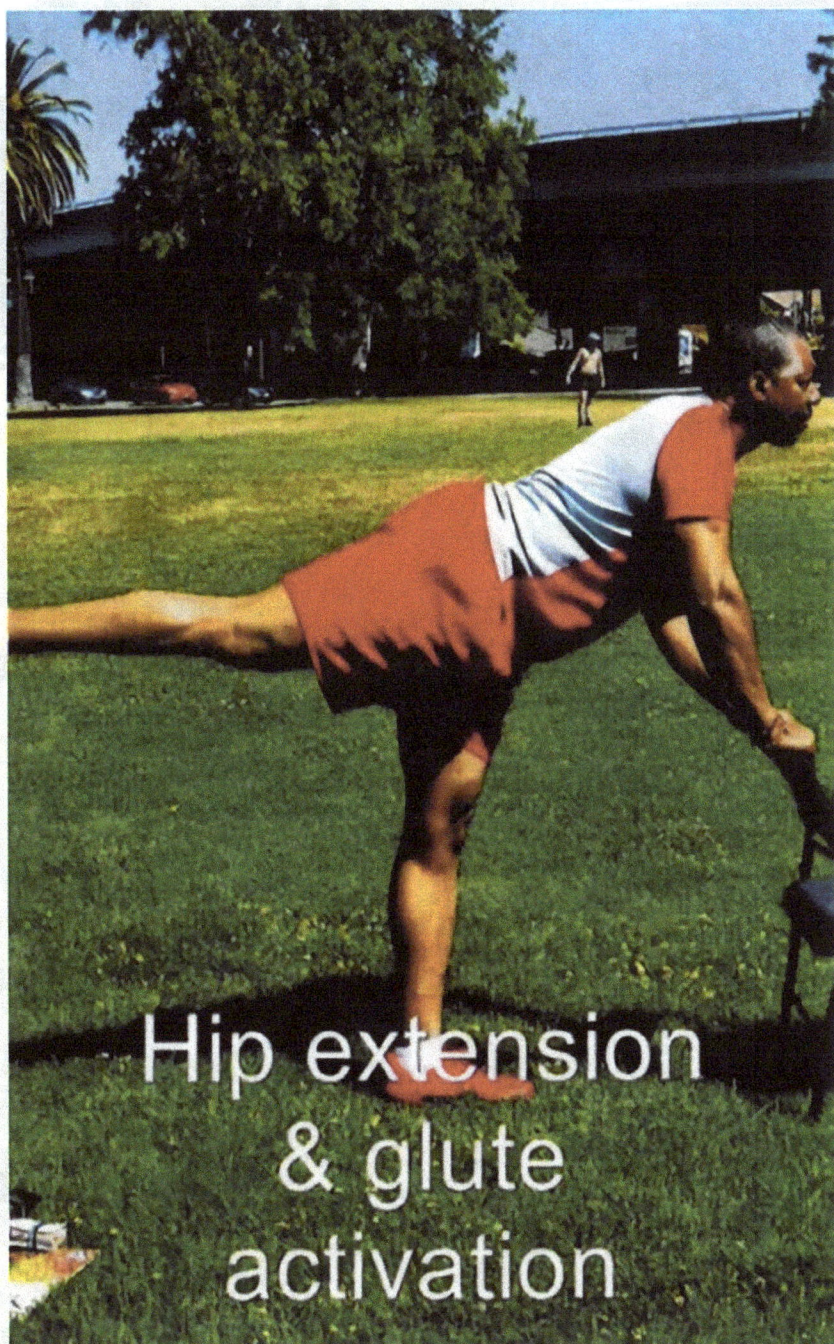

Hip extension
& glute
activation

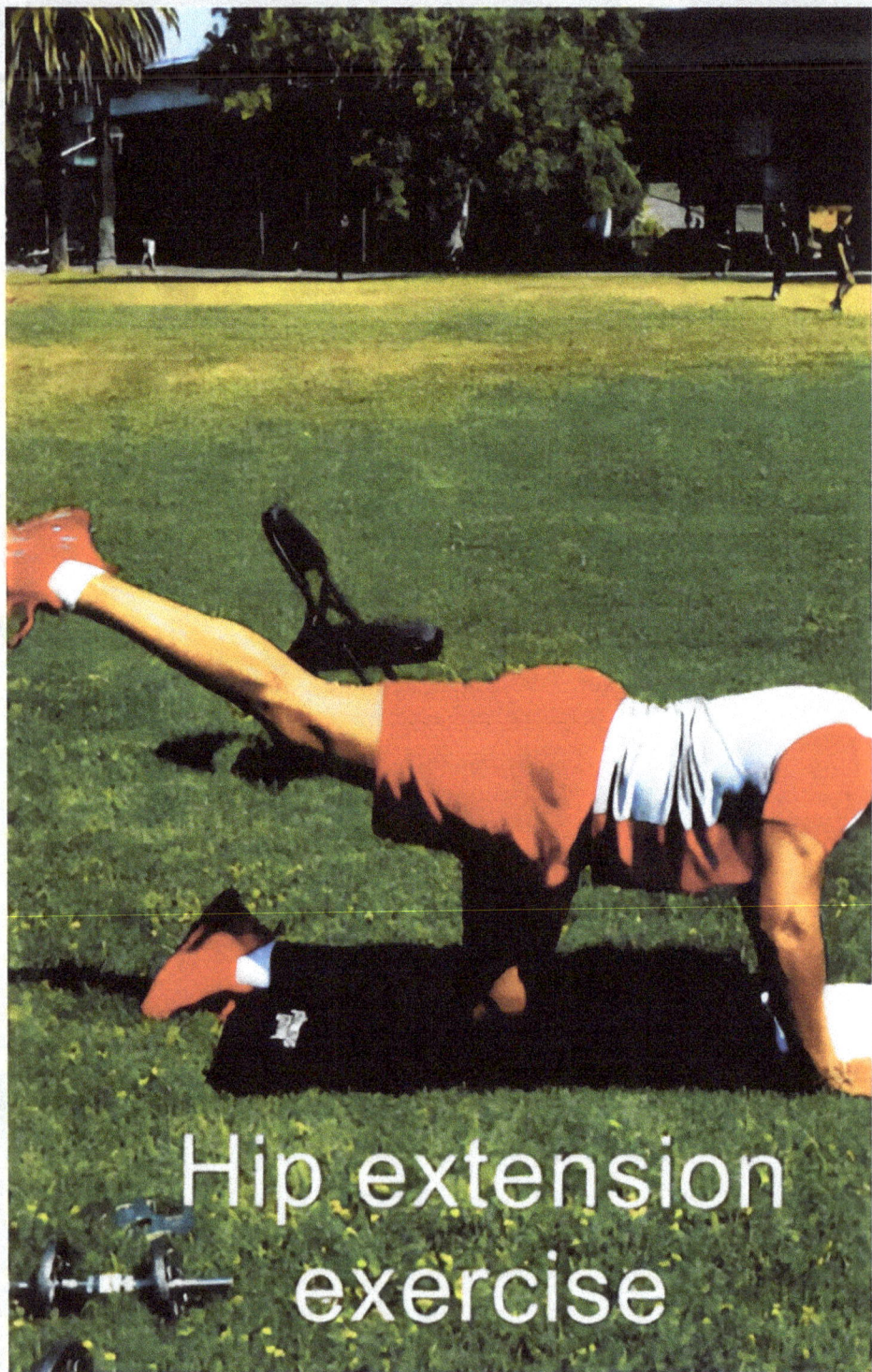

Hip extension exercise

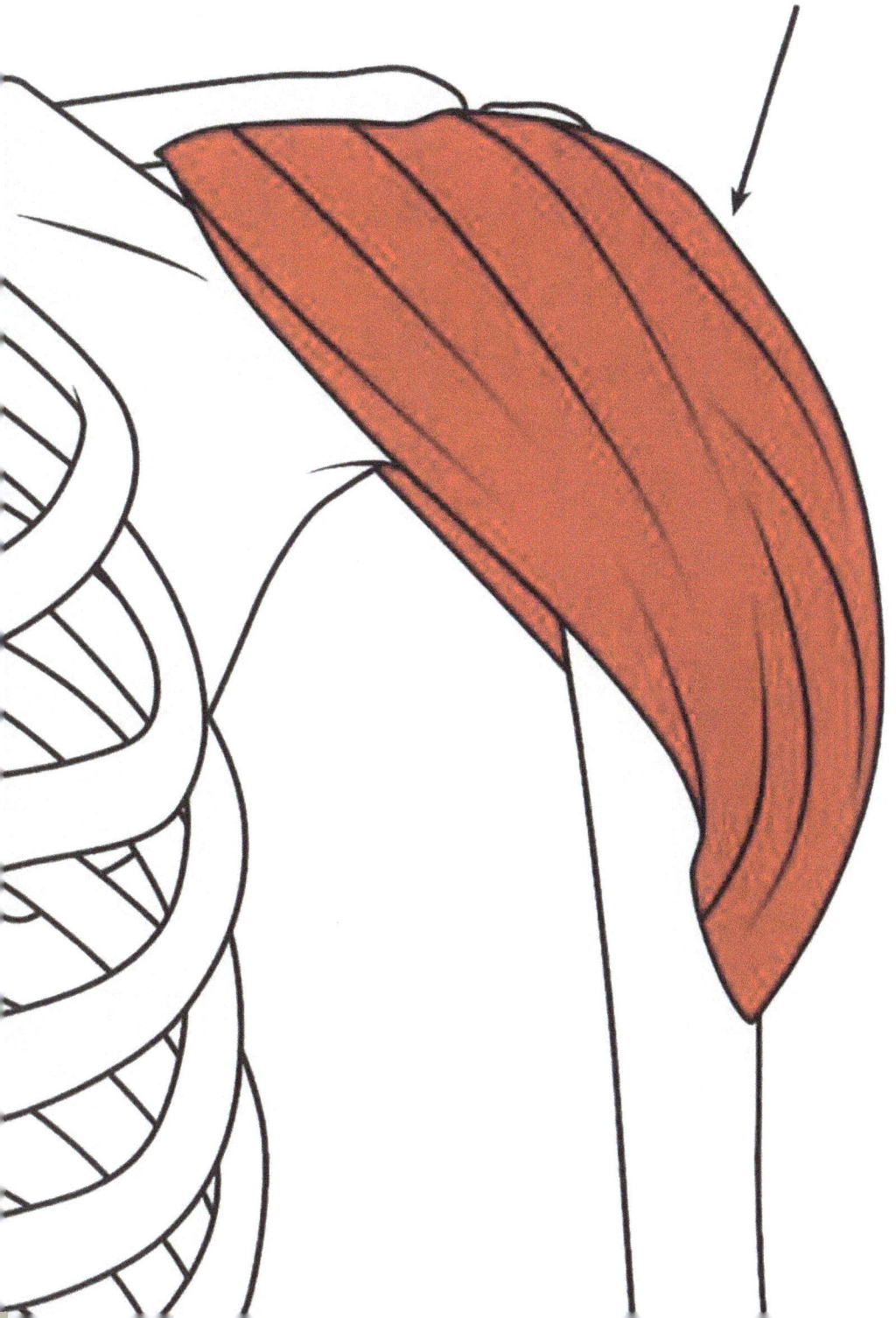

DELTOID

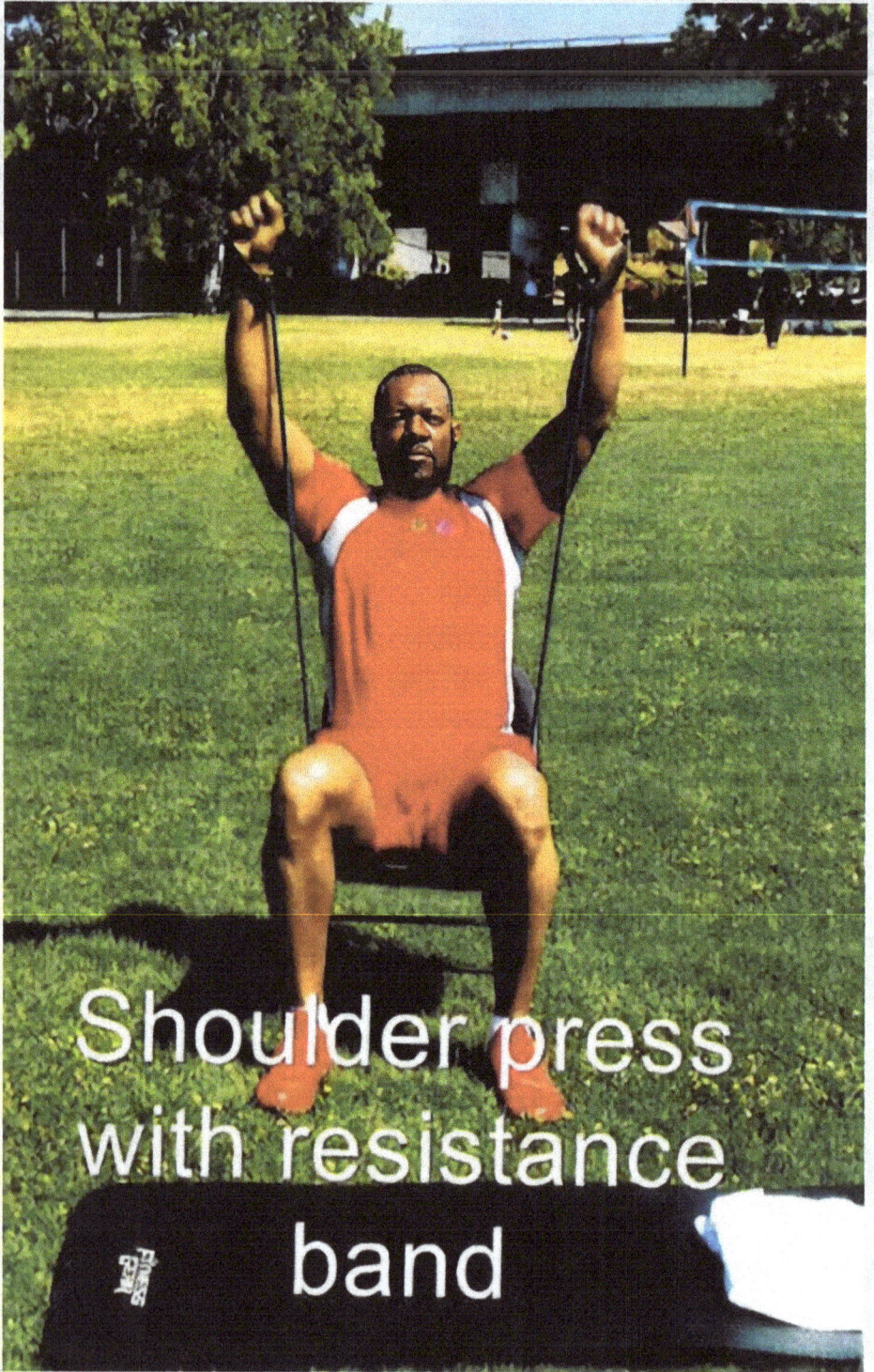

Shoulder press
with resistance
band

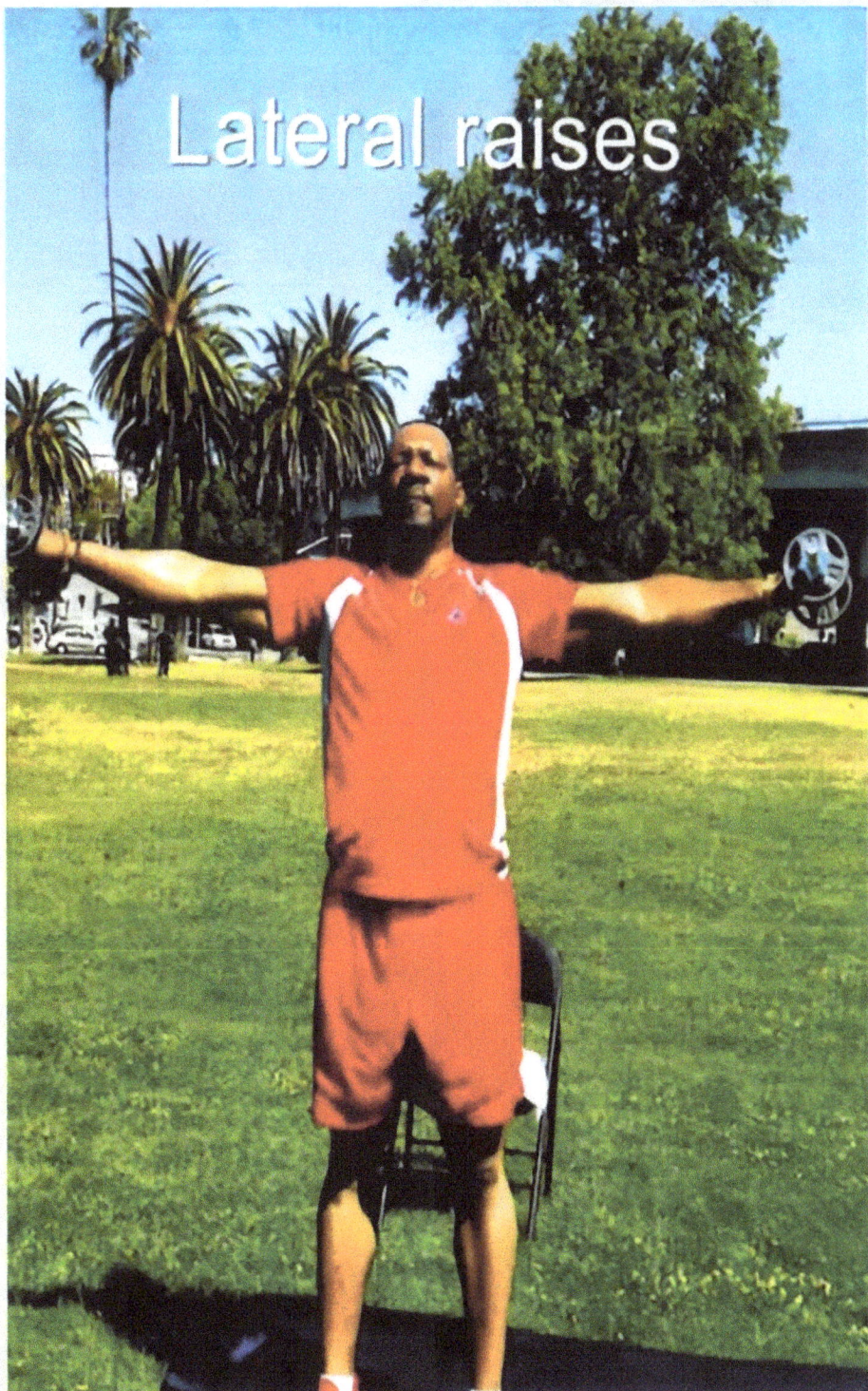

Lateral raises

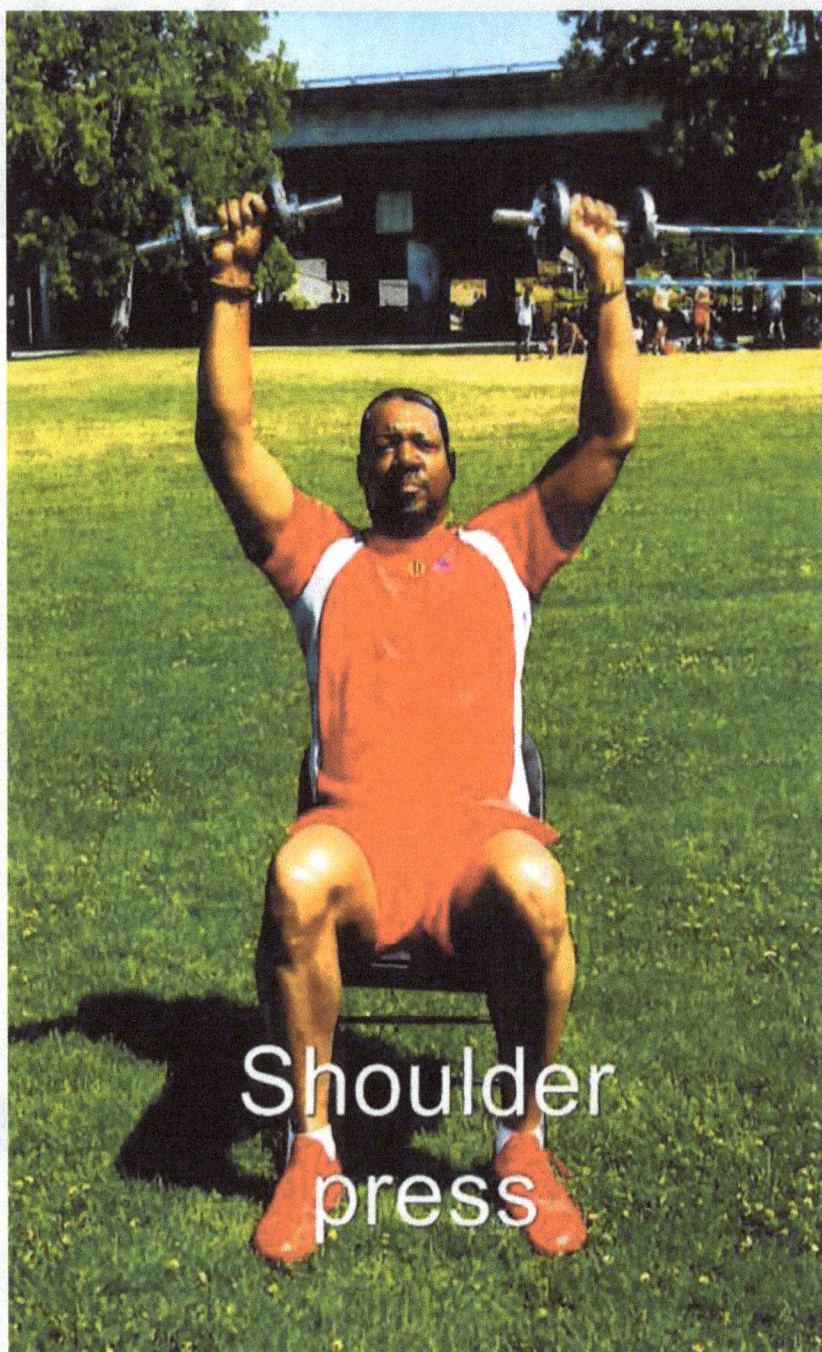

Shoulder press

I recommend exercising your shoulders with a resistance band of moderate tension or light to medium dumbbells. The effective exercises are lateral raises and shoulder presses in addition to external rotation of the humerus with a resistance band.

To avoid pain and injury to the deltoids when driving, always try to hold the steering wheel with both hands and palms up. Use the push-pull method.

This method will prevent shoulder injury. It is good for your posture.

Core Muscles

Core muscles spare the spine from heavy loads. They also core transfer force from the lower body to the upper body. Having a strong, stable core helps prevent injuries and allows us to perform at our optimum.

A poor sitting posture compromises the core. You need to engage your core in an upright posture whenever you are sitting. Tightening your stomach muscles while sitting can strengthen your core. A weak core causes back problems.

While operating a vehicle, the tight position is to tighten your stomach muscles, and sit tall and upright with the chest out and shoulders back. That will promote good posture and reduce the risk of injury.

The Trapezius

The Trapezius is a back muscle responsible for posture. It is used when tilting and turning the head and neck, shrugging, steadying the shoulders, and twisting the arms.

If you have shoulder and neck pain, it is very likely your posture is bad, and your Trapezius needs some attention as well as some exercise.

After driving for an hour, you need to get out of the seat and do some external rotations of the humerus. Use a resistance band of moderate tension.

The Knee

The knee joins the thigh bone (femur) to the shin bone (tibia). Sitting for long periods of time can cause knee pain.

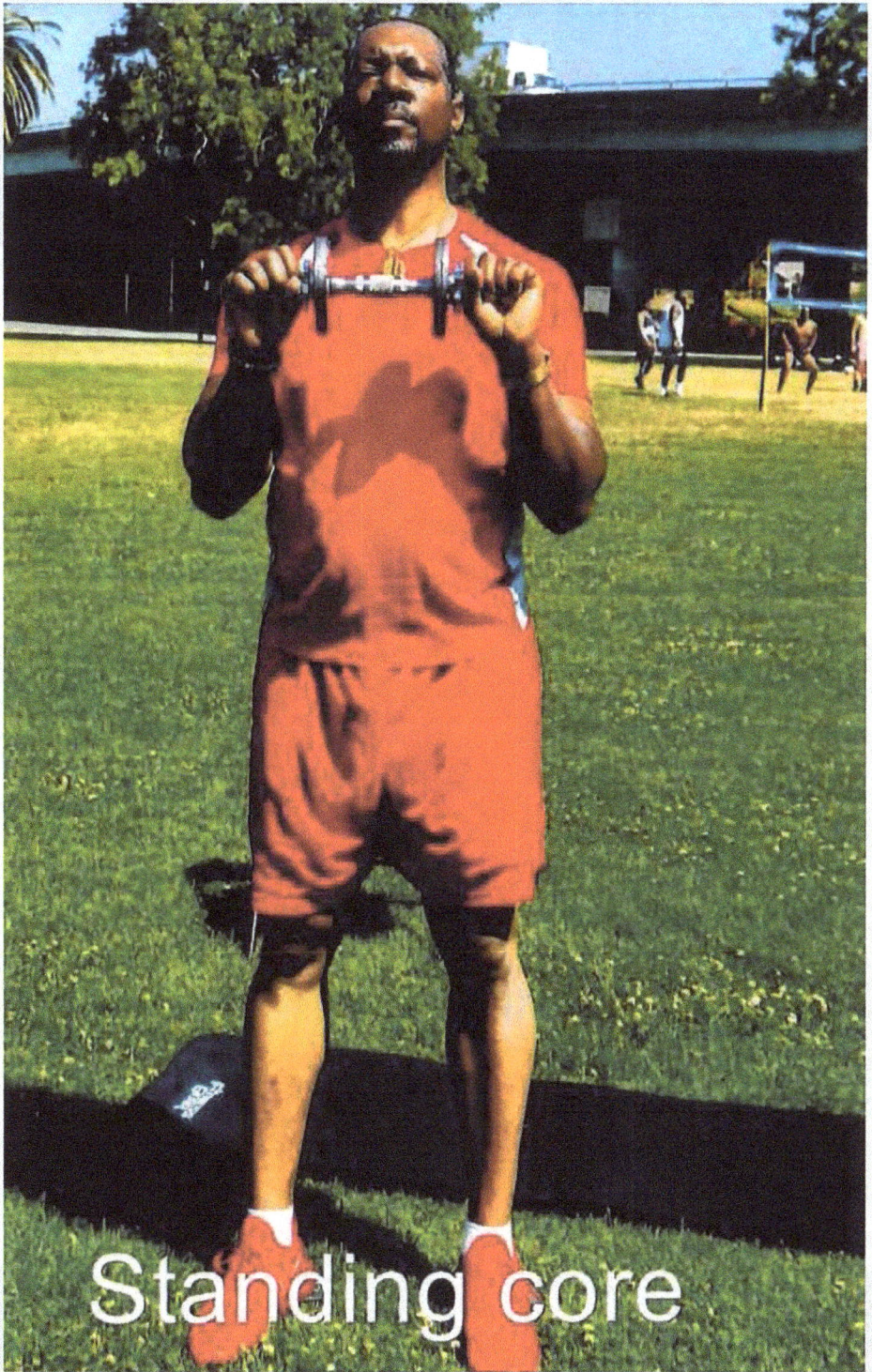

Standing core

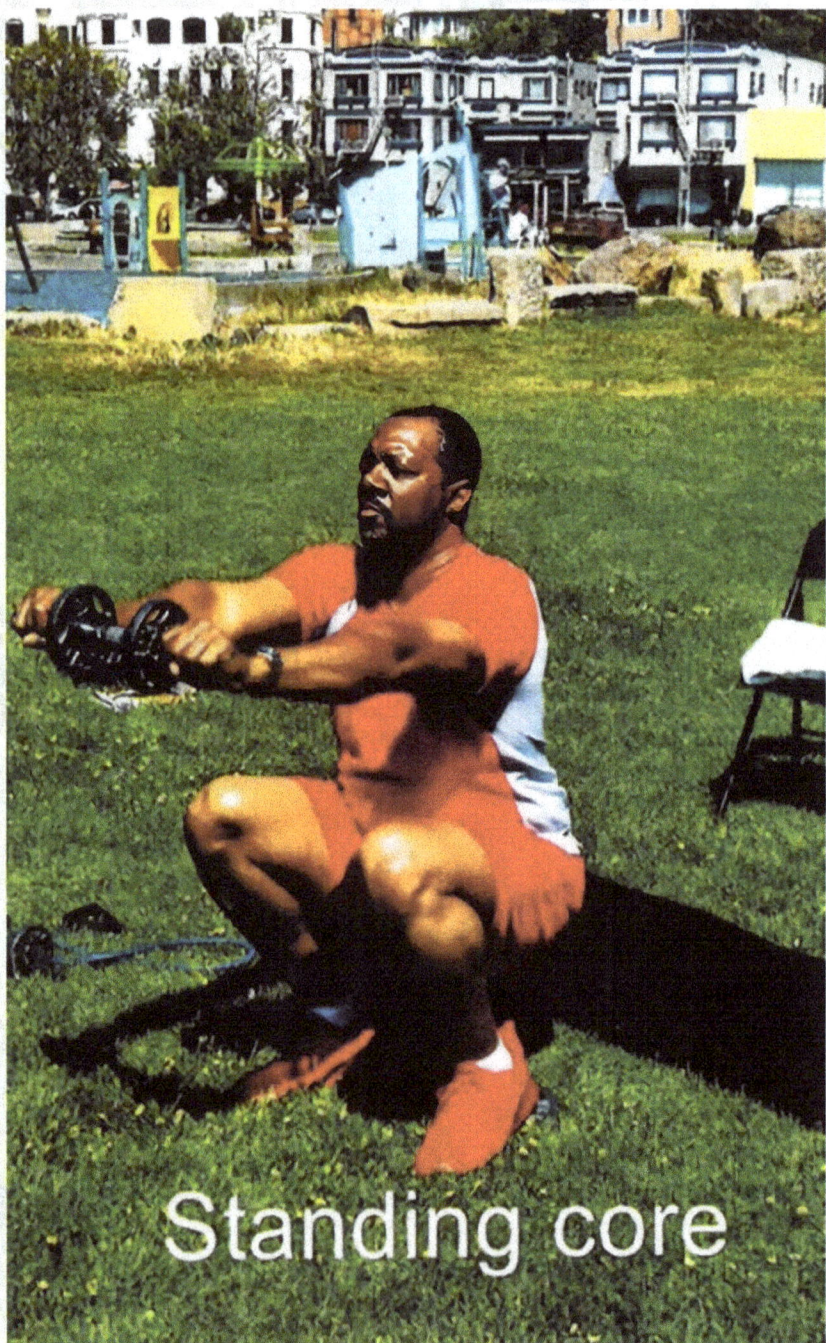

Standing core

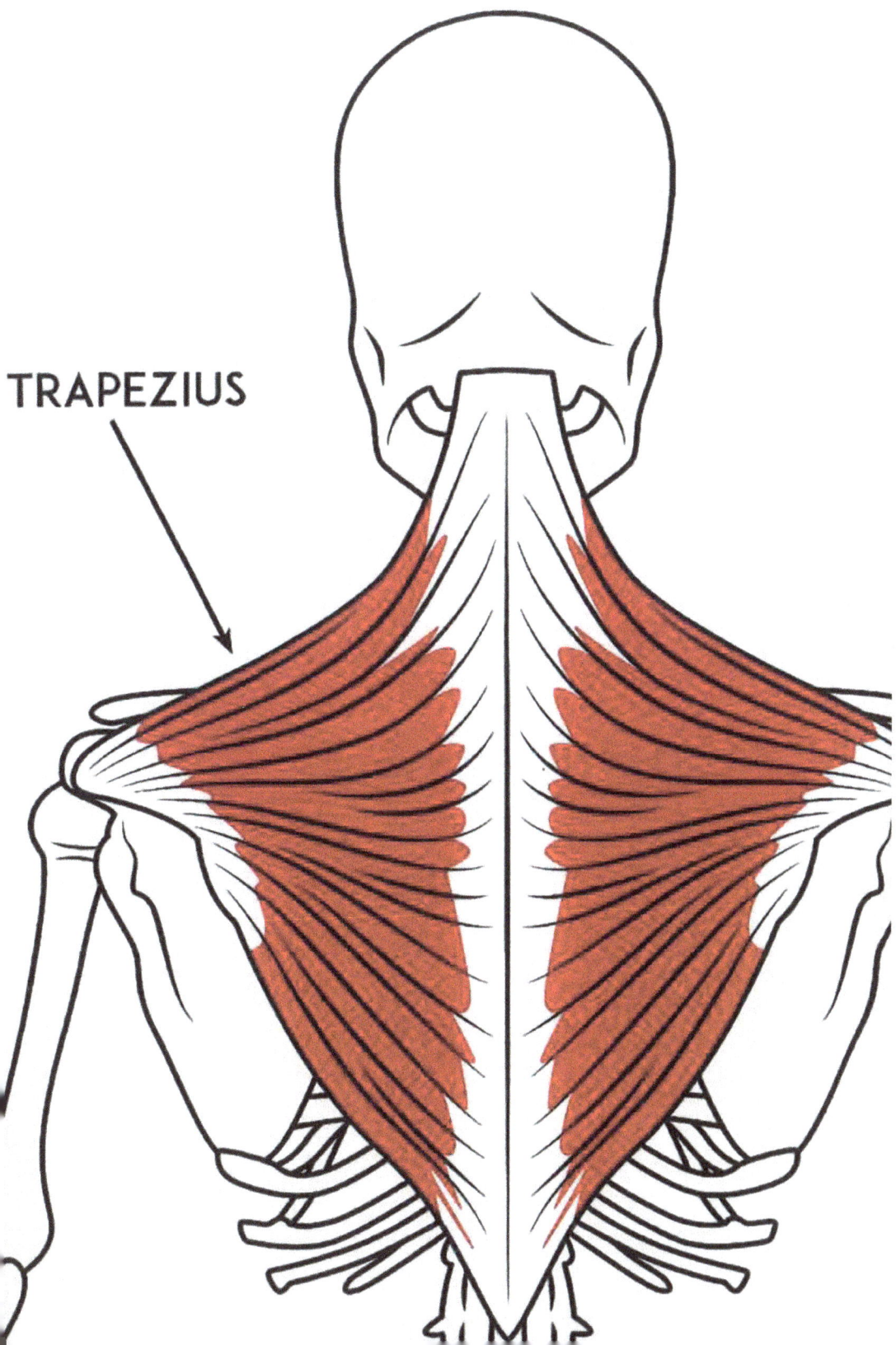

TRAPEZIUS

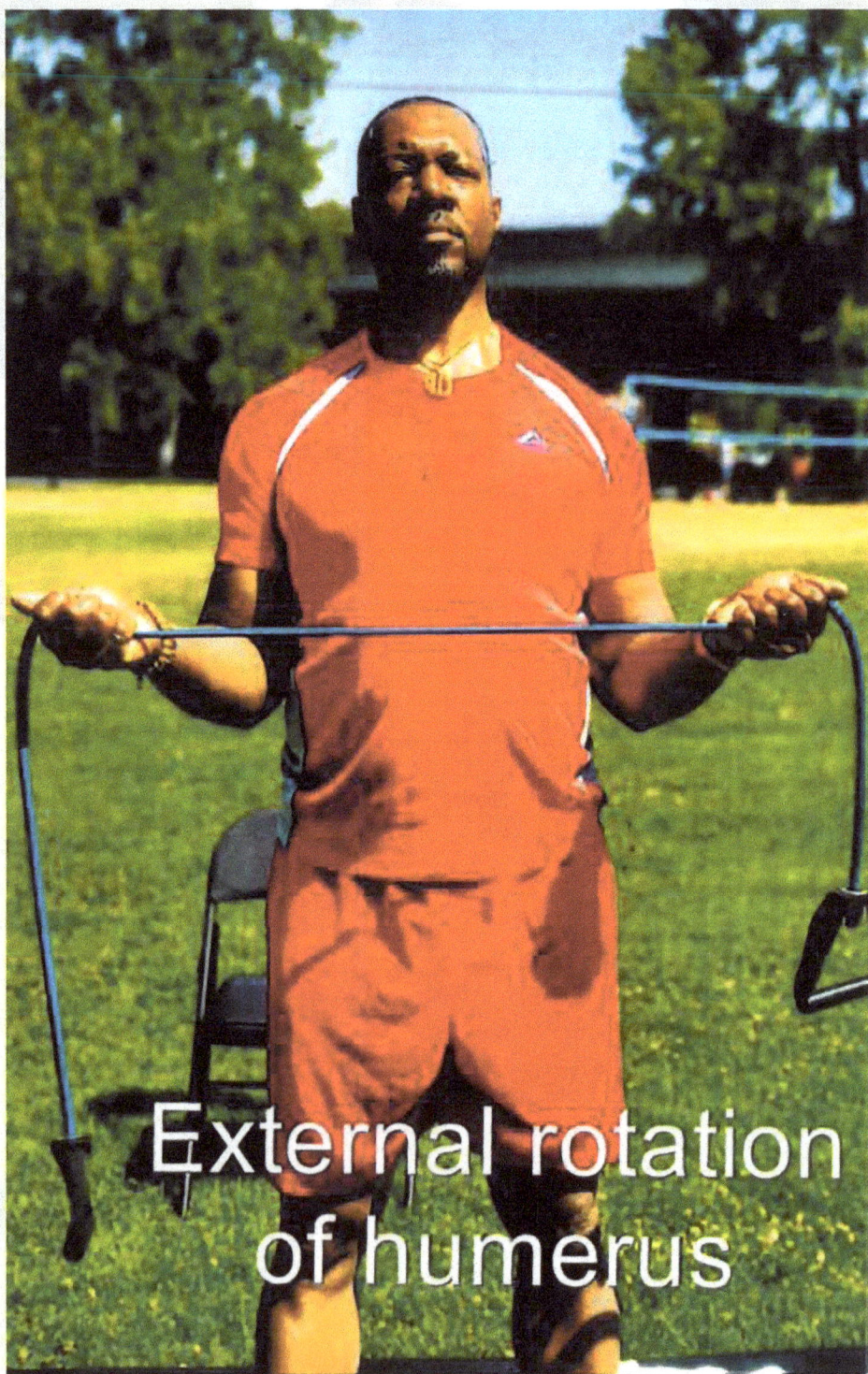

External rotation
of humerus

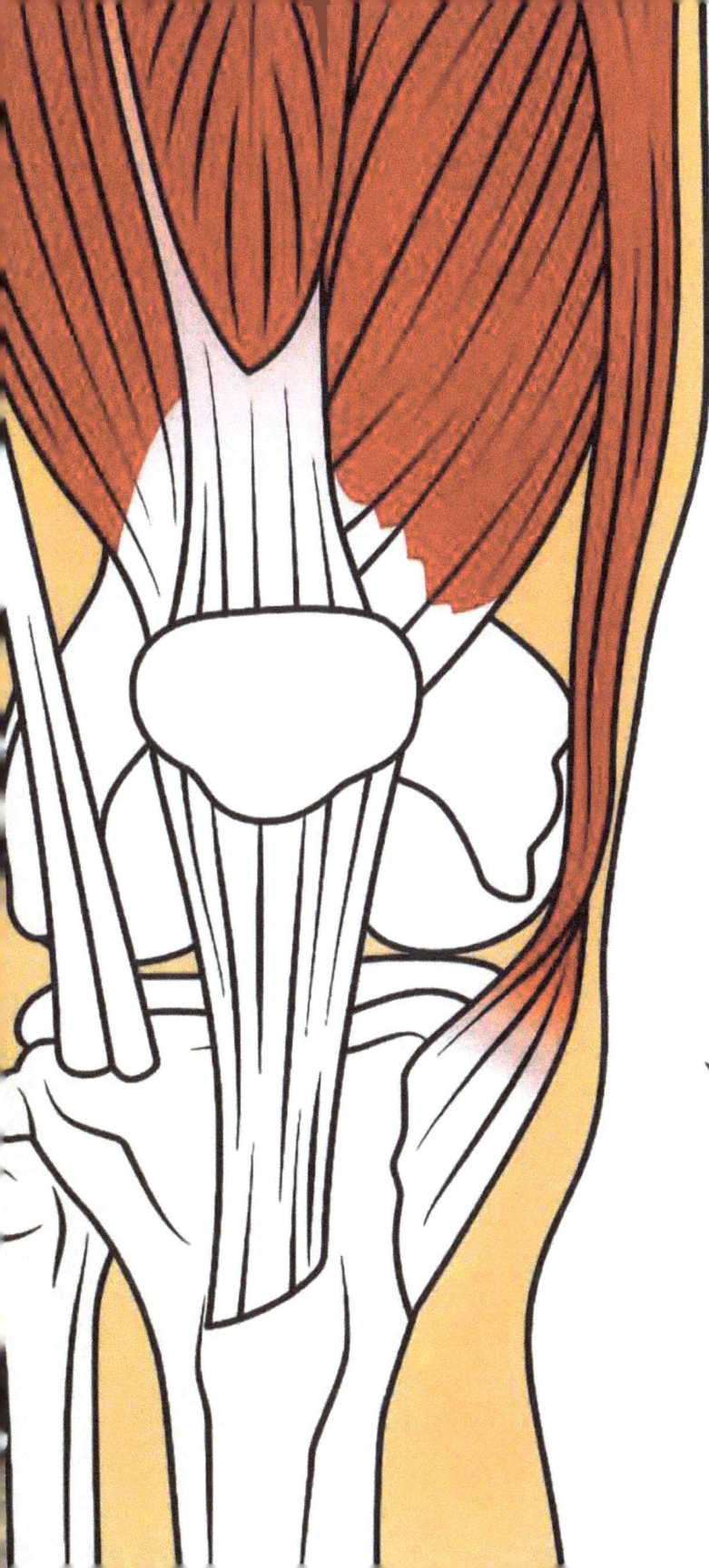

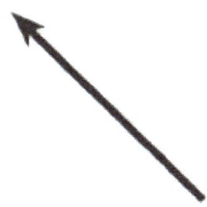

KNEE

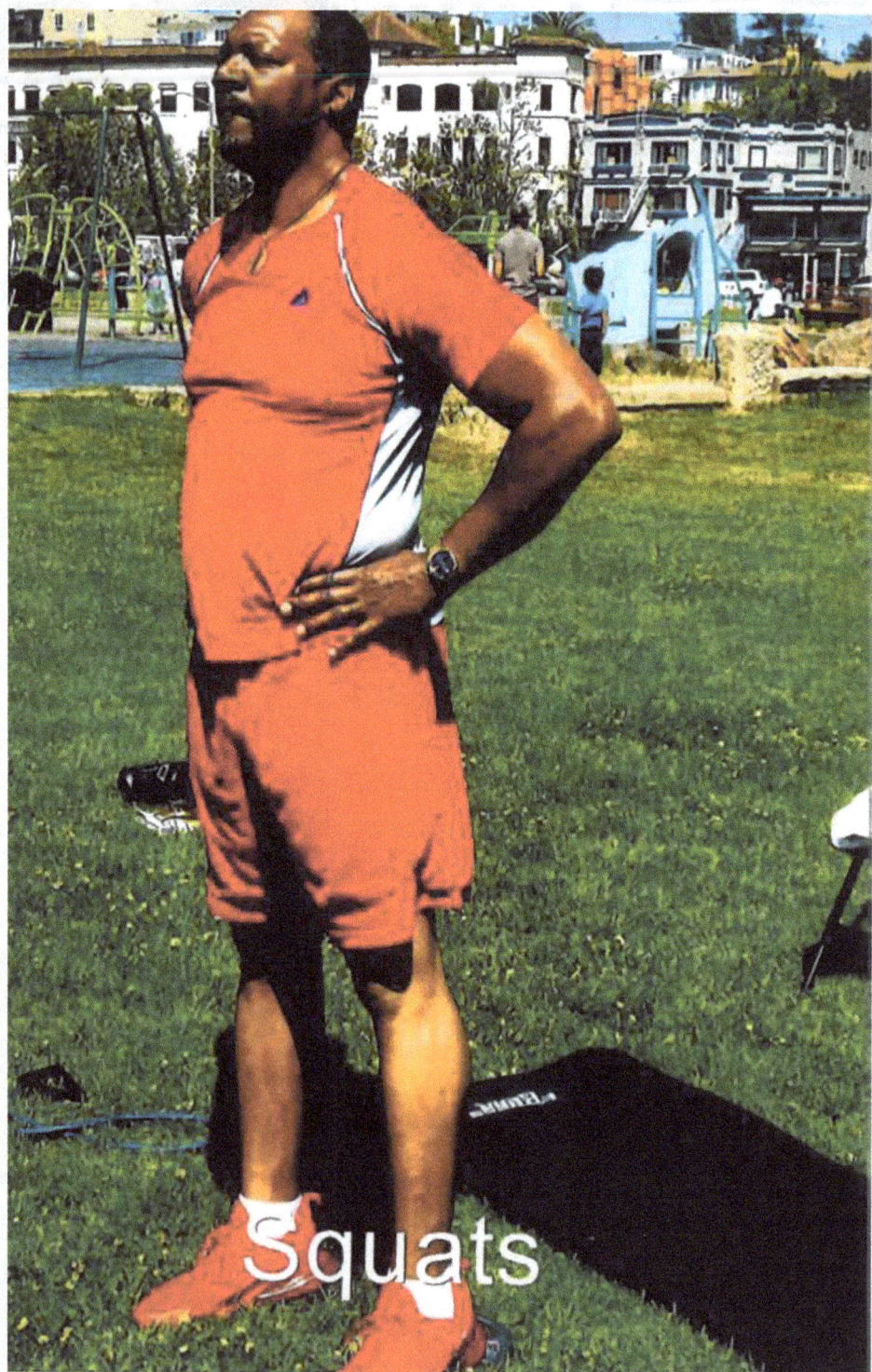

Squats

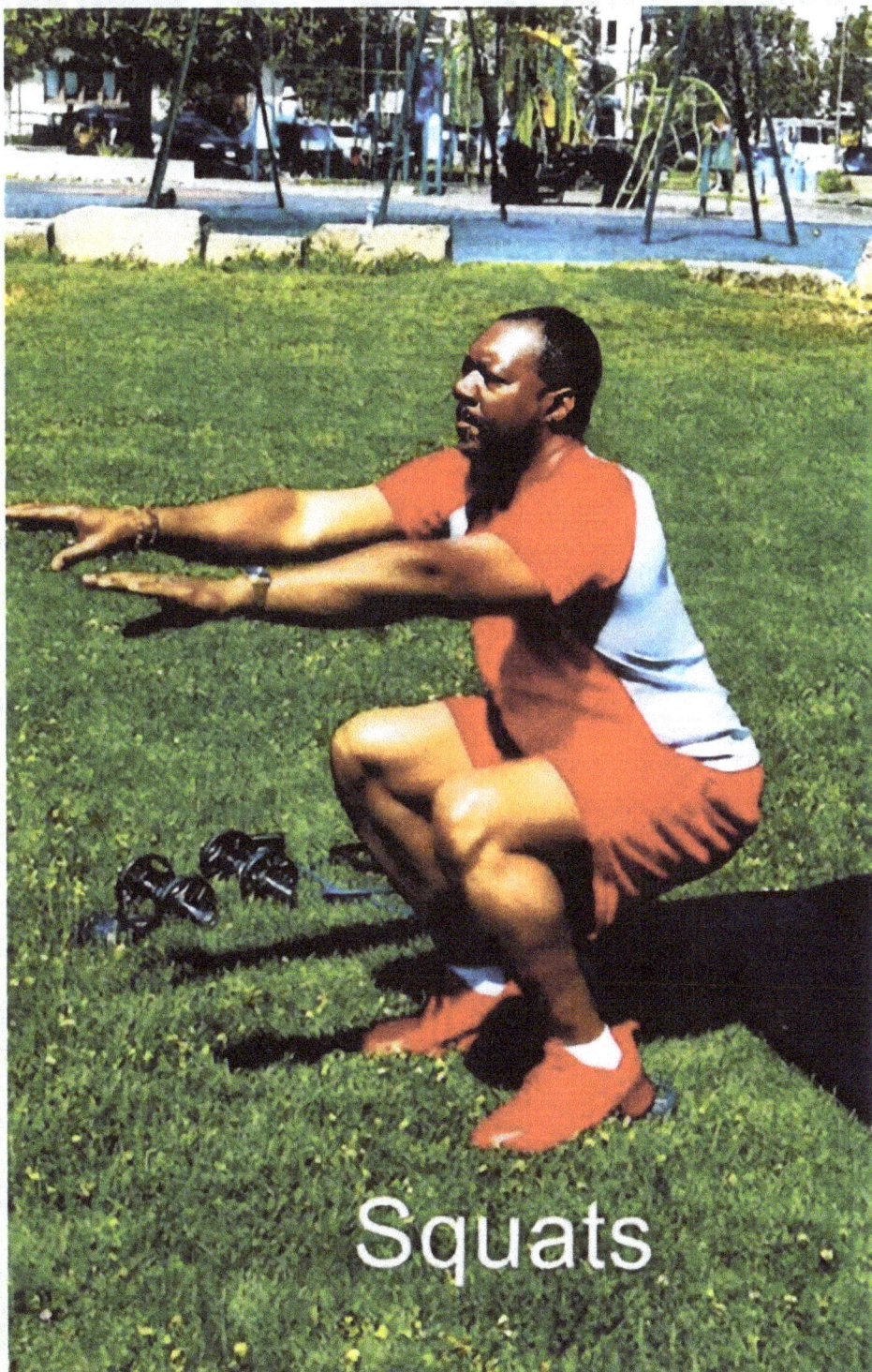

Squats

You need to get up and extend your knees frequently when driving, preferably after driving or sitting for an hour.

Squats and cycling are good exercises for the knee. Stretching every muscle attached to the knee will also help prevent injury to the knee.

The sedentary nature of driving is probably one of the reasons those who drive for a living have to make a concerted effort to fight off heart disease.

There are three things on the rise among commercial drivers: Diabetes, high blood pressure, and sleep apnea. Being overweight, having unhealthy eating habits, and not exercising contribute toward getting the big 3.

Stress is one of the things associated with commercial driving. Stress is a killer. One of the best ways to combat stress is a healthy lifestyle. For example, exercise, healthy eating, a positive attitude, and a hobby or outlet to help relieve stress. Medical professionals also recommend being active, as a career involving sitting for too long is like new cancer.

One way to burn calories, strengthen the heart, increase stamina and reduce stress is to do cardiovascular exercises. For example, brisk walking, swimming, using an elliptical machine, and cycling. When doing cardio exercises, pay attention to your heart rate. Your maximum heart rate is 220 bpm minus your age. To burn fat and not muscle, you want your heart rate between 60 percent and 80 percent of your maximum heart rate. If your heart rate is over 80 percent of your maximum heart rate for an extended period of time, you're at risk of burning muscle and fat.

> Example: 220bpm-age5o=170bpm is your heartrate
> I 70bpm x 60%=102bpm
> 170bpm x 80%=136bpm for a person age 50 to be in the fat burning zone, their heartrate should be between 102bpm and 136bpm

Nutrition is extremely important, especially to commercial drivers. Proper nutrition can help keep you healthy.

A plant-based diet has been proven to help people keep healthy and manage weight. Meal prep is also very helpful to a commercial driver. Having light, healthy meals or snacks with you while working will save you money and keep you healthy. Keep meals light and healthy while working so you don't get full, sleepy, and gassy.

Heat produces energy. Hot tea is another way to energize and soothe yourself while taking in little calories.

Ideal Meals Breakfast

Organic gluten-free oatmeal with blueberries and a small glass of orange juice.

Lunch: (Which should be the largest meal of the day)

Salad with chicken or shrimp (if eating out, soup and salad are excellent).

Dinner: Soup or salad, and of course, water throughout the day.

Mushrooms are an excellent meat substitute. Vegetables sauteed with mushrooms make a superb plant-based meal. You may want a carbohydrate with your meal. Wild rice is good. It's a whole grain and reduces the risk of heart disease. Another carb that is healthy and tasty is whole-grain pasta. When sauteing vegetables, olive oil with a little vegan butter is excellent.

THINGS TO CONSIDER

With so much traffic on the roads/highways and tight schedules, stress and anxiety can enter your day. Chamomile tea, ginger tea, and sleepy time tea all help with reducing stress and anxiety. They are also not addictive and are reasonably priced. They really have a calming effect and no side effects. I recommend these teas.

Breathing is an underrated, yet extremely important process. How you breathe can determine your heart rate, among other things. It is healthy and important to breathe and relax to bring down your heart rate. The brain needs oxygen for survival and proper functioning. Therefore, it is important to avoid holding your breath. In case you find you are breathing shallowly (breathing into your chest only), then you need to take a break. Sitting by a large body of water in nice weather would be ideal for you to relax and regain healthy breathing. Deep breaths are also good for your health.

Sleep is extremely important; it will rejuvenate you and keep your mood good. Lack of sleep makes you cranky, impatient, stressed, and clouds judgment. 8 hours of sleep a night is recommended.

Stretching is important and vital. It will keep you flexible.

Eating at least 28 grams of fiber a day is a good. It will help with the elimination process and help regulate blood sugar/blood pressure. Organic apples, organic carrots, organic broccoli, and gluten-free oatmeal are excellent sources of fiber.

Cinnamon may help regulate blood sugar.

White flour, white sugar, white rice, and white bread have no nutritional value, and contribute to inflammation in the body, which causes arthritis. In addition, it increases blood sugar.

Water is very vital. It hydrates the body, regulates body temperature, and helps eliminate waste. While driving, keep sipping your mountain spring water a little at a time. That will ensure it doesn't fill up your bladder fast.

I know some of you can manage or even function on alcohol and marijuana. However, they both impair your judgment and can affect your mood. Do not drink and drive or smoke/eat marijuana products while driving. A sober mind is a much sharper mind.

When driving, there is a good chance you will need to use the restroom. However, it may be a long way off. As a result, you have to hold it. That is one cause of a bladder infection.

Cranberry juice may help prevent urinary tract and bladder infections. Do not drink more than a liter a day.

Just like pain affects your blood pressure. Anxiety and stress affect your mood.

THINGS TO CONSIDER

Patience is a virtue and very much needed when sitting in standstill traffic. To ease your tension while sitting in traffic, think of future plans like a nice vacation.

I'm grateful to have worked 25 years and counting as a city bus operator. It's an honor and a privilege to serve the public.

If you're sitting an hour or more, sit on a cushion that keeps your tailbone from making contact with the seat. Further, try as much as possible to sit in alignment,; hips lined up with knees and knees lined up with your ankles.

This manual can greatly benefit new commercial drivers and anyone that sits long hours for a living. It can help you avoid some of the negative effects of your career.

I hope this manual benefits you in some way. Before you start any exercise program, consult a physician. By all means, try researching all the information in this manual.

The information in this manual is in addition to your physician's advice and any wellness department that works with your employer.

Thank you for taking time out of your life to read this manual. It has been a blessing to me, and I hope it's a blessing to you.

Remember, health is wealth. Robert T. Hancock

Important National Hotlines:

These are the hotlines you can call in case you need help with the following issues.

Substance Abuse: 1-800-662-HELP (4357) or TTY 1-800-487- 4889

Mental Health: 1-800-273-T ALK (8255)

Domestic Abuse: 1-800-799-7233 (SAFE) or 1-800-787-3224 (TTY)

Glossary

Achill Tendon
The fibrous cord connecting the calf and heel bone.

Anterior
The front part, near the front

Calf muscle
Muscles in the back portion of the lower leg.

Core muscles
Muscles of the torso

Deltoids
Thick triangular muscles covering the shoulder joint

Dumbbell
Short bar with weights on either end used for muscle-building exercises

Extension
Muscle movement that takes two body parts further from each other

Femur
Thigh bone between the hip and knee

Flexion
Muscle movement that brings two body parts closer to each other

Glutes
Buttock muscles

Hamstring
Tendons at the back of the knee

Heart rate
Number of heartbeats in a minute

Heel
Back part of the foot below the ankle

Hip flexors
Group of thigh muscles that facilitate flexing of the hip

Humerus
Upper arm bone from the shoulder to the elbow

Nutrition
Food or nourishment

Posterior
Back part/near the back

Quadriceps
Large front thigh muscle

Resistance band
The elastic band used for strength training

Sedentary
Inactive, sitting for long

Spine
Series of vertebrae from the skull to the small of the back providing support for the body; backbone

Tail bone
Arrangement of bones at the base of the spine

Tibia

The larger inner bone between the knee and ankle

Torso

The central part of the body

Trapezius

The large superficial back muscle that aids the movement of the neck, head, shoulders, and arms

ENDORSEMENT

"The health information contained within is valuable to not only commercial drivers, but in general to any human being who sits for long periods of time be it in the workplace or outside of it.

The visual illustrations are fun, bright and colorful and serve as a user-friendly guide for one to follow and execute the exercises designed to strengthen the muscles in question—those muscles that are most prone to weakness due to the (physically) repetitive lifestyles of the majority of human beings."

~ Norlisha Long, CNMT/LMT/HE **OMNI Health & Body Therapy/ NoLo F.I.R.M. Well-Fit**
Oakland/Alameda East Bay Area

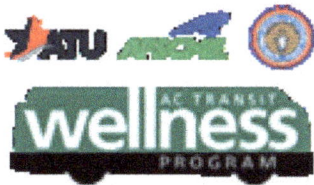

www.ingramcontent.com/pod-product-compliance
Lightning Source LLC
Chambersburg PA
CBHW052123030426
42335CB00025B/3089